WORKOUT LOG

NAME: _______________________ GOALS: _______________________

EXERCISES	SETS	REPS	WT	REST	TIME	1 RM	NOTES

DATE: __________ WEIGHT: __________ SLEEP: __________ CALORIES: __________

EXERCISES	SETS	REPS	WT	REST	TIME	1 RM	NOTES

DATE: __________ WEIGHT: __________ SLEEP: __________ CALORIES: __________

EXERCISES	SETS	REPS	WT	REST	TIME	1 RM	NOTES

DATE: __________ WEIGHT: __________ SLEEP: __________ CALORIES: __________

EXERCISES	SETS	REPS	WT	REST	TIME	1 RM	NOTES

DATE: __________ WEIGHT: __________ SLEEP: __________ CALORIES: __________

EXERCISES	SETS	REPS	WT	REST	TIME	1 RM	NOTES

DATE: __________ WEIGHT: __________ SLEEP: __________ CALORIES: __________

WORKOUT LOG

NAME:___________________________ GOALS:___________________________

EXERCISES	SETS	REPS	WT	REST	TIME	1 RM	NOTES

DATE:___________ WEIGHT:___________ SLEEP:___________ CALORIES:___________

EXERCISES	SETS	REPS	WT	REST	TIME	1 RM	NOTES

DATE:___________ WEIGHT:___________ SLEEP:___________ CALORIES:___________

EXERCISES	SETS	REPS	WT	REST	TIME	1 RM	NOTES

DATE:___________ WEIGHT:___________ SLEEP:___________ CALORIES:___________

EXERCISES	SETS	REPS	WT	REST	TIME	1 RM	NOTES

DATE:___________ WEIGHT:___________ SLEEP:___________ CALORIES:___________

EXERCISES	SETS	REPS	WT	REST	TIME	1 RM	NOTES

DATE:___________ WEIGHT:___________ SLEEP:___________ CALORIES:___________

WORKOUT LOG

NAME:_____________________________ GOALS:_____________________________

EXERCISES	SETS	REPS	WT	REST	TIME	1 RM	NOTES

DATE:__________ WEIGHT:__________ SLEEP:__________ CALORIES:__________

EXERCISES	SETS	REPS	WT	REST	TIME	1 RM	NOTES

DATE:__________ WEIGHT:__________ SLEEP:__________ CALORIES:__________

EXERCISES	SETS	REPS	WT	REST	TIME	1 RM	NOTES

DATE:__________ WEIGHT:__________ SLEEP:__________ CALORIES:__________

EXERCISES	SETS	REPS	WT	REST	TIME	1 RM	NOTES

DATE:__________ WEIGHT:__________ SLEEP:__________ CALORIES:__________

EXERCISES	SETS	REPS	WT	REST	TIME	1 RM	NOTES

DATE:__________ WEIGHT:__________ SLEEP:__________ CALORIES:__________

WORKOUT LOG

NAME:________________________   GOALS:________________________

EXERCISES	SETS	REPS	WT	REST	TIME	1 RM	NOTES

DATE:__________   WEIGHT:__________   SLEEP:__________   CALORIES:__________

EXERCISES	SETS	REPS	WT	REST	TIME	1 RM	NOTES

DATE:__________   WEIGHT:__________   SLEEP:__________   CALORIES:__________

EXERCISES	SETS	REPS	WT	REST	TIME	1 RM	NOTES

DATE:__________   WEIGHT:__________   SLEEP:__________   CALORIES:__________

EXERCISES	SETS	REPS	WT	REST	TIME	1 RM	NOTES

DATE:__________   WEIGHT:__________   SLEEP:__________   CALORIES:__________

EXERCISES	SETS	REPS	WT	REST	TIME	1 RM	NOTES

DATE:__________   WEIGHT:__________   SLEEP:__________   CALORIES:__________

WORKOUT LOG

NAME:_________________________ GOALS:_________________________

EXERCISES	SETS	REPS	WT	REST	TIME	1 RM	NOTES

DATE:__________ WEIGHT:__________ SLEEP:__________ CALORIES:__________

EXERCISES	SETS	REPS	WT	REST	TIME	1 RM	NOTES

DATE:__________ WEIGHT:__________ SLEEP:__________ CALORIES:__________

EXERCISES	SETS	REPS	WT	REST	TIME	1 RM	NOTES

DATE:__________ WEIGHT:__________ SLEEP:__________ CALORIES:__________

EXERCISES	SETS	REPS	WT	REST	TIME	1 RM	NOTES

DATE:__________ WEIGHT:__________ SLEEP:__________ CALORIES:__________

EXERCISES	SETS	REPS	WT	REST	TIME	1 RM	NOTES

DATE:__________ WEIGHT:__________ SLEEP:__________ CALORIES:__________

WORKOUT LOG

NAME:________________________ GOALS:________________________

EXERCISES	SETS	REPS	WT	REST	TIME	1 RM	NOTES

DATE:__________ WEIGHT:__________ SLEEP:__________ CALORIES:__________

EXERCISES	SETS	REPS	WT	REST	TIME	1 RM	NOTES

DATE:__________ WEIGHT:__________ SLEEP:__________ CALORIES:__________

EXERCISES	SETS	REPS	WT	REST	TIME	1 RM	NOTES

DATE:__________ WEIGHT:__________ SLEEP:__________ CALORIES:__________

EXERCISES	SETS	REPS	WT	REST	TIME	1 RM	NOTES

DATE:__________ WEIGHT:__________ SLEEP:__________ CALORIES:__________

EXERCISES	SETS	REPS	WT	REST	TIME	1 RM	NOTES

DATE:__________ WEIGHT:__________ SLEEP:__________ CALORIES:__________

WORKOUT LOG

NAME:______________________   GOALS:______________________

EXERCISES	SETS	REPS	WT	REST	TIME	1 RM	NOTES

DATE:__________   WEIGHT:__________   SLEEP:__________   CALORIES:__________

EXERCISES	SETS	REPS	WT	REST	TIME	1 RM	NOTES

DATE:__________   WEIGHT:__________   SLEEP:__________   CALORIES:__________

EXERCISES	SETS	REPS	WT	REST	TIME	1 RM	NOTES

DATE:__________   WEIGHT:__________   SLEEP:__________   CALORIES:__________

EXERCISES	SETS	REPS	WT	REST	TIME	1 RM	NOTES

DATE:__________   WEIGHT:__________   SLEEP:__________   CALORIES:__________

EXERCISES	SETS	REPS	WT	REST	TIME	1 RM	NOTES

DATE:__________   WEIGHT:__________   SLEEP:__________   CALORIES:__________

WORKOUT LOG

NAME:________________________ GOALS:________________________

EXERCISES	SETS	REPS	WT	REST	TIME	1 RM	NOTES

DATE:__________ WEIGHT:__________ SLEEP:__________ CALORIES:__________

EXERCISES	SETS	REPS	WT	REST	TIME	1 RM	NOTES

DATE:__________ WEIGHT:__________ SLEEP:__________ CALORIES:__________

EXERCISES	SETS	REPS	WT	REST	TIME	1 RM	NOTES

DATE:__________ WEIGHT:__________ SLEEP:__________ CALORIES:__________

EXERCISES	SETS	REPS	WT	REST	TIME	1 RM	NOTES

DATE:__________ WEIGHT:__________ SLEEP:__________ CALORIES:__________

EXERCISES	SETS	REPS	WT	REST	TIME	1 RM	NOTES

DATE:__________ WEIGHT:__________ SLEEP:__________ CALORIES:__________

WORKOUT LOG

NAME:_____________________   GOALS:_____________________

EXERCISES	SETS	REPS	WT	REST	TIME	1 RM	NOTES

DATE:_________   WEIGHT:_________   SLEEP:_________   CALORIES:_________

EXERCISES	SETS	REPS	WT	REST	TIME	1 RM	NOTES

DATE:_________   WEIGHT:_________   SLEEP:_________   CALORIES:_________

EXERCISES	SETS	REPS	WT	REST	TIME	1 RM	NOTES

DATE:_________   WEIGHT:_________   SLEEP:_________   CALORIES:_________

EXERCISES	SETS	REPS	WT	REST	TIME	1 RM	NOTES

DATE:_________   WEIGHT:_________   SLEEP:_________   CALORIES:_________

EXERCISES	SETS	REPS	WT	REST	TIME	1 RM	NOTES

DATE:_________   WEIGHT:_________   SLEEP:_________   CALORIES:_________

WORKOUT LOG

NAME:______________________________ GOALS:______________________________

EXERCISES	SETS	REPS	WT	REST	TIME	1 RM	NOTES

DATE:__________   WEIGHT:__________   SLEEP:__________   CALORIES:__________

EXERCISES	SETS	REPS	WT	REST	TIME	1 RM	NOTES

DATE:__________   WEIGHT:__________   SLEEP:__________   CALORIES:__________

EXERCISES	SETS	REPS	WT	REST	TIME	1 RM	NOTES

DATE:__________   WEIGHT:__________   SLEEP:__________   CALORIES:__________

EXERCISES	SETS	REPS	WT	REST	TIME	1 RM	NOTES

DATE:__________   WEIGHT:__________   SLEEP:__________   CALORIES:__________

EXERCISES	SETS	REPS	WT	REST	TIME	1 RM	NOTES

DATE:__________   WEIGHT:__________   SLEEP:__________   CALORIES:__________

WORKOUT LOG

NAME:___________________________ GOALS:____________________________

EXERCISES	SETS	REPS	WT	REST	TIME	1 RM	NOTES

DATE:___________ WEIGHT:___________ SLEEP:___________ CALORIES:___________

EXERCISES	SETS	REPS	WT	REST	TIME	1 RM	NOTES

DATE:___________ WEIGHT:___________ SLEEP:___________ CALORIES:___________

EXERCISES	SETS	REPS	WT	REST	TIME	1 RM	NOTES

DATE:___________ WEIGHT:___________ SLEEP:___________ CALORIES:___________

EXERCISES	SETS	REPS	WT	REST	TIME	1 RM	NOTES

DATE:___________ WEIGHT:___________ SLEEP:___________ CALORIES:___________

EXERCISES	SETS	REPS	WT	REST	TIME	1 RM	NOTES

DATE:___________ WEIGHT:___________ SLEEP:___________ CALORIES:___________

WORKOUT LOG

NAME:_________________________ GOALS:_____________________

EXERCISES	SETS	REPS	WT	REST	TIME	1 RM	NOTES

DATE:_________ WEIGHT:_________ SLEEP:_________ CALORIES:_________

EXERCISES	SETS	REPS	WT	REST	TIME	1 RM	NOTES

DATE:_________ WEIGHT:_________ SLEEP:_________ CALORIES:_________

EXERCISES	SETS	REPS	WT	REST	TIME	1 RM	NOTES

DATE:_________ WEIGHT:_________ SLEEP:_________ CALORIES:_________

EXERCISES	SETS	REPS	WT	REST	TIME	1 RM	NOTES

DATE:_________ WEIGHT:_________ SLEEP:_________ CALORIES:_________

EXERCISES	SETS	REPS	WT	REST	TIME	1 RM	NOTES

DATE:_________ WEIGHT:_________ SLEEP:_________ CALORIES:_________

WORKOUT LOG

NAME:__________________________   GOALS:__________________________

EXERCISES	SETS	REPS	WT	REST	TIME	1 RM	NOTES

DATE:__________   WEIGHT:__________   SLEEP:__________   CALORIES:__________

EXERCISES	SETS	REPS	WT	REST	TIME	1 RM	NOTES

DATE:__________   WEIGHT:__________   SLEEP:__________   CALORIES:__________

EXERCISES	SETS	REPS	WT	REST	TIME	1 RM	NOTES

DATE:__________   WEIGHT:__________   SLEEP:__________   CALORIES:__________

EXERCISES	SETS	REPS	WT	REST	TIME	1 RM	NOTES

DATE:__________   WEIGHT:__________   SLEEP:__________   CALORIES:__________

EXERCISES	SETS	REPS	WT	REST	TIME	1 RM	NOTES

DATE:__________   WEIGHT:__________   SLEEP:__________   CALORIES:__________

WORKOUT LOG

NAME:________________________   GOALS:________________________

EXERCISES	SETS	REPS	WT	REST	TIME	1 RM	NOTES

DATE:__________   WEIGHT:__________   SLEEP:__________   CALORIES:__________

EXERCISES	SETS	REPS	WT	REST	TIME	1 RM	NOTES

DATE:__________   WEIGHT:__________   SLEEP:__________   CALORIES:__________

EXERCISES	SETS	REPS	WT	REST	TIME	1 RM	NOTES

DATE:__________   WEIGHT:__________   SLEEP:__________   CALORIES:__________

EXERCISES	SETS	REPS	WT	REST	TIME	1 RM	NOTES

DATE:__________   WEIGHT:__________   SLEEP:__________   CALORIES:__________

EXERCISES	SETS	REPS	WT	REST	TIME	1 RM	NOTES

DATE:__________   WEIGHT:__________   SLEEP:__________   CALORIES:__________

WORKOUT LOG

NAME:_________________________ GOALS:_________________________

EXERCISES	SETS	REPS	WT	REST	TIME	1 RM	NOTES

DATE:__________   WEIGHT:__________   SLEEP:__________   CALORIES:__________

EXERCISES	SETS	REPS	WT	REST	TIME	1 RM	NOTES

DATE:__________   WEIGHT:__________   SLEEP:__________   CALORIES:__________

EXERCISES	SETS	REPS	WT	REST	TIME	1 RM	NOTES

DATE:__________   WEIGHT:__________   SLEEP:__________   CALORIES:__________

EXERCISES	SETS	REPS	WT	REST	TIME	1 RM	NOTES

DATE:__________   WEIGHT:__________   SLEEP:__________   CALORIES:__________

EXERCISES	SETS	REPS	WT	REST	TIME	1 RM	NOTES

DATE:__________   WEIGHT:__________   SLEEP:__________   CALORIES:__________

WORKOUT LOG

NAME:_________________________ GOALS:_________________________

EXERCISES	SETS	REPS	WT	REST	TIME	1 RM	NOTES

DATE:_________ WEIGHT:_________ SLEEP:_________ CALORIES:_________

EXERCISES	SETS	REPS	WT	REST	TIME	1 RM	NOTES

DATE:_________ WEIGHT:_________ SLEEP:_________ CALORIES:_________

EXERCISES	SETS	REPS	WT	REST	TIME	1 RM	NOTES

DATE:_________ WEIGHT:_________ SLEEP:_________ CALORIES:_________

EXERCISES	SETS	REPS	WT	REST	TIME	1 RM	NOTES

DATE:_________ WEIGHT:_________ SLEEP:_________ CALORIES:_________

EXERCISES	SETS	REPS	WT	REST	TIME	1 RM	NOTES

DATE:_________ WEIGHT:_________ SLEEP:_________ CALORIES:_________

WORKOUT LOG

NAME:__________________________   GOALS:__________________________

EXERCISES	SETS	REPS	WT	REST	TIME	1 RM	NOTES

DATE:__________   WEIGHT:__________   SLEEP:__________   CALORIES:__________

EXERCISES	SETS	REPS	WT	REST	TIME	1 RM	NOTES

DATE:__________   WEIGHT:__________   SLEEP:__________   CALORIES:__________

EXERCISES	SETS	REPS	WT	REST	TIME	1 RM	NOTES

DATE:__________   WEIGHT:__________   SLEEP:__________   CALORIES:__________

EXERCISES	SETS	REPS	WT	REST	TIME	1 RM	NOTES

DATE:__________   WEIGHT:__________   SLEEP:__________   CALORIES:__________

EXERCISES	SETS	REPS	WT	REST	TIME	1 RM	NOTES

DATE:__________   WEIGHT:__________   SLEEP:__________   CALORIES:__________

WORKOUT LOG

NAME:______________________________   GOALS:____________________________

EXERCISES	SETS	REPS	WT	REST	TIME	1 RM	NOTES

DATE:__________   WEIGHT:__________   SLEEP:__________   CALORIES:__________

EXERCISES	SETS	REPS	WT	REST	TIME	1 RM	NOTES

DATE:__________   WEIGHT:__________   SLEEP:__________   CALORIES:__________

EXERCISES	SETS	REPS	WT	REST	TIME	1 RM	NOTES

DATE:__________   WEIGHT:__________   SLEEP:__________   CALORIES:__________

EXERCISES	SETS	REPS	WT	REST	TIME	1 RM	NOTES

DATE:__________   WEIGHT:__________   SLEEP:__________   CALORIES:__________

EXERCISES	SETS	REPS	WT	REST	TIME	1 RM	NOTES

DATE:__________   WEIGHT:__________   SLEEP:__________   CALORIES:__________

WORKOUT LOG

NAME:_______________________ GOALS:_______________________

EXERCISES	SETS	REPS	WT	REST	TIME	1 RM	NOTES

DATE:__________ WEIGHT:__________ SLEEP:__________ CALORIES:__________

EXERCISES	SETS	REPS	WT	REST	TIME	1 RM	NOTES

DATE:__________ WEIGHT:__________ SLEEP:__________ CALORIES:__________

EXERCISES	SETS	REPS	WT	REST	TIME	1 RM	NOTES

DATE:__________ WEIGHT:__________ SLEEP:__________ CALORIES:__________

EXERCISES	SETS	REPS	WT	REST	TIME	1 RM	NOTES

DATE:__________ WEIGHT:__________ SLEEP:__________ CALORIES:__________

EXERCISES	SETS	REPS	WT	REST	TIME	1 RM	NOTES

DATE:__________ WEIGHT:__________ SLEEP:__________ CALORIES:__________

WORKOUT LOG

NAME:___________________________ GOALS:___________________________

EXERCISES	SETS	REPS	WT	REST	TIME	1 RM	NOTES

DATE:__________ WEIGHT:__________ SLEEP:__________ CALORIES:__________

EXERCISES	SETS	REPS	WT	REST	TIME	1 RM	NOTES

DATE:__________ WEIGHT:__________ SLEEP:__________ CALORIES:__________

EXERCISES	SETS	REPS	WT	REST	TIME	1 RM	NOTES

DATE:__________ WEIGHT:__________ SLEEP:__________ CALORIES:__________

EXERCISES	SETS	REPS	WT	REST	TIME	1 RM	NOTES

DATE:__________ WEIGHT:__________ SLEEP:__________ CALORIES:__________

EXERCISES	SETS	REPS	WT	REST	TIME	1 RM	NOTES

DATE:__________ WEIGHT:__________ SLEEP:__________ CALORIES:__________

WORKOUT LOG

NAME:_________________________   GOALS:_________________________

EXERCISES	SETS	REPS	WT	REST	TIME	1 RM	NOTES

DATE:__________   WEIGHT:__________   SLEEP:__________   CALORIES:__________

EXERCISES	SETS	REPS	WT	REST	TIME	1 RM	NOTES

DATE:__________   WEIGHT:__________   SLEEP:__________   CALORIES:__________

EXERCISES	SETS	REPS	WT	REST	TIME	1 RM	NOTES

DATE:__________   WEIGHT:__________   SLEEP:__________   CALORIES:__________

EXERCISES	SETS	REPS	WT	REST	TIME	1 RM	NOTES

DATE:__________   WEIGHT:__________   SLEEP:__________   CALORIES:__________

EXERCISES	SETS	REPS	WT	REST	TIME	1 RM	NOTES

DATE:__________   WEIGHT:__________   SLEEP:__________   CALORIES:__________

WORKOUT LOG

NAME:________________________   GOALS:________________________

EXERCISES	SETS	REPS	WT	REST	TIME	1 RM	NOTES

DATE:__________   WEIGHT:__________   SLEEP:__________   CALORIES:__________

EXERCISES	SETS	REPS	WT	REST	TIME	1 RM	NOTES

DATE:__________   WEIGHT:__________   SLEEP:__________   CALORIES:__________

EXERCISES	SETS	REPS	WT	REST	TIME	1 RM	NOTES

DATE:__________   WEIGHT:__________   SLEEP:__________   CALORIES:__________

EXERCISES	SETS	REPS	WT	REST	TIME	1 RM	NOTES

DATE:__________   WEIGHT:__________   SLEEP:__________   CALORIES:__________

EXERCISES	SETS	REPS	WT	REST	TIME	1 RM	NOTES

DATE:__________   WEIGHT:__________   SLEEP:__________   CALORIES:__________

WORKOUT LOG

NAME: _______________________   GOALS: _______________________

EXERCISES	SETS	REPS	WT	REST	TIME	1 RM	NOTES

DATE: __________   WEIGHT: __________   SLEEP: __________   CALORIES: __________

EXERCISES	SETS	REPS	WT	REST	TIME	1 RM	NOTES

DATE: __________   WEIGHT: __________   SLEEP: __________   CALORIES: __________

EXERCISES	SETS	REPS	WT	REST	TIME	1 RM	NOTES

DATE: __________   WEIGHT: __________   SLEEP: __________   CALORIES: __________

EXERCISES	SETS	REPS	WT	REST	TIME	1 RM	NOTES

DATE: __________   WEIGHT: __________   SLEEP: __________   CALORIES: __________

EXERCISES	SETS	REPS	WT	REST	TIME	1 RM	NOTES

DATE: __________   WEIGHT: __________   SLEEP: __________   CALORIES: __________

WORKOUT LOG

NAME:_________________________   GOALS:_________________________

EXERCISES	SETS	REPS	WT	REST	TIME	1 RM	NOTES

DATE:_________   WEIGHT:_________   SLEEP:_________   CALORIES:_________

EXERCISES	SETS	REPS	WT	REST	TIME	1 RM	NOTES

DATE:_________   WEIGHT:_________   SLEEP:_________   CALORIES:_________

EXERCISES	SETS	REPS	WT	REST	TIME	1 RM	NOTES

DATE:_________   WEIGHT:_________   SLEEP:_________   CALORIES:_________

EXERCISES	SETS	REPS	WT	REST	TIME	1 RM	NOTES

DATE:_________   WEIGHT:_________   SLEEP:_________   CALORIES:_________

EXERCISES	SETS	REPS	WT	REST	TIME	1 RM	NOTES

DATE:_________   WEIGHT:_________   SLEEP:_________   CALORIES:_________

WORKOUT LOG

NAME:_________________________   GOALS:_________________________

EXERCISES	SETS	REPS	WT	REST	TIME	1 RM	NOTES

DATE:_________   WEIGHT:_________   SLEEP:_________   CALORIES:_________

EXERCISES	SETS	REPS	WT	REST	TIME	1 RM	NOTES

DATE:_________   WEIGHT:_________   SLEEP:_________   CALORIES:_________

EXERCISES	SETS	REPS	WT	REST	TIME	1 RM	NOTES

DATE:_________   WEIGHT:_________   SLEEP:_________   CALORIES:_________

EXERCISES	SETS	REPS	WT	REST	TIME	1 RM	NOTES

DATE:_________   WEIGHT:_________   SLEEP:_________   CALORIES:_________

EXERCISES	SETS	REPS	WT	REST	TIME	1 RM	NOTES

DATE:_________   WEIGHT:_________   SLEEP:_________   CALORIES:_________

WORKOUT LOG

NAME:__________________________ GOALS:__________________________

EXERCISES	SETS	REPS	WT	REST	TIME	1 RM	NOTES

DATE:__________   WEIGHT:__________   SLEEP:__________   CALORIES:__________

EXERCISES	SETS	REPS	WT	REST	TIME	1 RM	NOTES

DATE:__________   WEIGHT:__________   SLEEP:__________   CALORIES:__________

EXERCISES	SETS	REPS	WT	REST	TIME	1 RM	NOTES

DATE:__________   WEIGHT:__________   SLEEP:__________   CALORIES:__________

EXERCISES	SETS	REPS	WT	REST	TIME	1 RM	NOTES

DATE:__________   WEIGHT:__________   SLEEP:__________   CALORIES:__________

EXERCISES	SETS	REPS	WT	REST	TIME	1 RM	NOTES

DATE:__________   WEIGHT:__________   SLEEP:__________   CALORIES:__________

WORKOUT LOG

NAME:________________________ GOALS:________________________

EXERCISES	SETS	REPS	WT	REST	TIME	1 RM	NOTES

DATE:__________ WEIGHT:__________ SLEEP:__________ CALORIES:__________

EXERCISES	SETS	REPS	WT	REST	TIME	1 RM	NOTES

DATE:__________ WEIGHT:__________ SLEEP:__________ CALORIES:__________

EXERCISES	SETS	REPS	WT	REST	TIME	1 RM	NOTES

DATE:__________ WEIGHT:__________ SLEEP:__________ CALORIES:__________

EXERCISES	SETS	REPS	WT	REST	TIME	1 RM	NOTES

DATE:__________ WEIGHT:__________ SLEEP:__________ CALORIES:__________

EXERCISES	SETS	REPS	WT	REST	TIME	1 RM	NOTES

DATE:__________ WEIGHT:__________ SLEEP:__________ CALORIES:__________

WORKOUT LOG

NAME:____________________   GOALS:____________________

EXERCISES	SETS	REPS	WT	REST	TIME	1 RM	NOTES

DATE:__________   WEIGHT:__________   SLEEP:__________   CALORIES:__________

EXERCISES	SETS	REPS	WT	REST	TIME	1 RM	NOTES

DATE:__________   WEIGHT:__________   SLEEP:__________   CALORIES:__________

EXERCISES	SETS	REPS	WT	REST	TIME	1 RM	NOTES

DATE:__________   WEIGHT:__________   SLEEP:__________   CALORIES:__________

EXERCISES	SETS	REPS	WT	REST	TIME	1 RM	NOTES

DATE:__________   WEIGHT:__________   SLEEP:__________   CALORIES:__________

EXERCISES	SETS	REPS	WT	REST	TIME	1 RM	NOTES

DATE:__________   WEIGHT:__________   SLEEP:__________   CALORIES:__________

WORKOUT LOG

NAME:_________________________   GOALS:_________________________

EXERCISES	SETS	REPS	WT	REST	TIME	1 RM	NOTES

DATE:_________   WEIGHT:_________   SLEEP:_________   CALORIES:_________

EXERCISES	SETS	REPS	WT	REST	TIME	1 RM	NOTES

DATE:_________   WEIGHT:_________   SLEEP:_________   CALORIES:_________

EXERCISES	SETS	REPS	WT	REST	TIME	1 RM	NOTES

DATE:_________   WEIGHT:_________   SLEEP:_________   CALORIES:_________

EXERCISES	SETS	REPS	WT	REST	TIME	1 RM	NOTES

DATE:_________   WEIGHT:_________   SLEEP:_________   CALORIES:_________

EXERCISES	SETS	REPS	WT	REST	TIME	1 RM	NOTES

DATE:_________   WEIGHT:_________   SLEEP:_________   CALORIES:_________

WORKOUT LOG

NAME:_________________________ GOALS:_________________________

EXERCISES	SETS	REPS	WT	REST	TIME	1 RM	NOTES

DATE:__________   WEIGHT:__________   SLEEP:__________   CALORIES:__________

EXERCISES	SETS	REPS	WT	REST	TIME	1 RM	NOTES

DATE:__________   WEIGHT:__________   SLEEP:__________   CALORIES:__________

EXERCISES	SETS	REPS	WT	REST	TIME	1 RM	NOTES

DATE:__________   WEIGHT:__________   SLEEP:__________   CALORIES:__________

EXERCISES	SETS	REPS	WT	REST	TIME	1 RM	NOTES

DATE:__________   WEIGHT:__________   SLEEP:__________   CALORIES:__________

EXERCISES	SETS	REPS	WT	REST	TIME	1 RM	NOTES

DATE:__________   WEIGHT:__________   SLEEP:__________   CALORIES:__________

WORKOUT LOG

NAME:________________________ GOALS:___________________________

EXERCISES	SETS	REPS	WT	REST	TIME	1 RM	NOTES

DATE:__________ WEIGHT:__________ SLEEP:__________ CALORIES:__________

EXERCISES	SETS	REPS	WT	REST	TIME	1 RM	NOTES

DATE:__________ WEIGHT:__________ SLEEP:__________ CALORIES:__________

EXERCISES	SETS	REPS	WT	REST	TIME	1 RM	NOTES

DATE:__________ WEIGHT:__________ SLEEP:__________ CALORIES:__________

EXERCISES	SETS	REPS	WT	REST	TIME	1 RM	NOTES

DATE:__________ WEIGHT:__________ SLEEP:__________ CALORIES:__________

EXERCISES	SETS	REPS	WT	REST	TIME	1 RM	NOTES

DATE:__________ WEIGHT:__________ SLEEP:__________ CALORIES:__________

WORKOUT LOG

NAME:__________________________   GOALS:__________________________

EXERCISES	SETS	REPS	WT	REST	TIME	1 RM	NOTES

DATE:__________   WEIGHT:__________   SLEEP:__________   CALORIES:__________

EXERCISES	SETS	REPS	WT	REST	TIME	1 RM	NOTES

DATE:__________   WEIGHT:__________   SLEEP:__________   CALORIES:__________

EXERCISES	SETS	REPS	WT	REST	TIME	1 RM	NOTES

DATE:__________   WEIGHT:__________   SLEEP:__________   CALORIES:__________

EXERCISES	SETS	REPS	WT	REST	TIME	1 RM	NOTES

DATE:__________   WEIGHT:__________   SLEEP:__________   CALORIES:__________

EXERCISES	SETS	REPS	WT	REST	TIME	1 RM	NOTES

DATE:__________   WEIGHT:__________   SLEEP:__________   CALORIES:__________

WORKOUT LOG

NAME:_________________________   GOALS:_____________________

EXERCISES	SETS	REPS	WT	REST	TIME	1 RM	NOTES

DATE:__________   WEIGHT:__________   SLEEP:__________   CALORIES:__________

EXERCISES	SETS	REPS	WT	REST	TIME	1 RM	NOTES

DATE:__________   WEIGHT:__________   SLEEP:__________   CALORIES:__________

EXERCISES	SETS	REPS	WT	REST	TIME	1 RM	NOTES

DATE:__________   WEIGHT:__________   SLEEP:__________   CALORIES:__________

EXERCISES	SETS	REPS	WT	REST	TIME	1 RM	NOTES

DATE:__________   WEIGHT:__________   SLEEP:__________   CALORIES:__________

EXERCISES	SETS	REPS	WT	REST	TIME	1 RM	NOTES

DATE:__________   WEIGHT:__________   SLEEP:__________   CALORIES:__________

WORKOUT LOG

NAME:________________________   GOALS:________________________

EXERCISES	SETS	REPS	WT	REST	TIME	1 RM	NOTES

DATE:__________   WEIGHT:__________   SLEEP:__________   CALORIES:__________

EXERCISES	SETS	REPS	WT	REST	TIME	1 RM	NOTES

DATE:__________   WEIGHT:__________   SLEEP:__________   CALORIES:__________

EXERCISES	SETS	REPS	WT	REST	TIME	1 RM	NOTES

DATE:__________   WEIGHT:__________   SLEEP:__________   CALORIES:__________

EXERCISES	SETS	REPS	WT	REST	TIME	1 RM	NOTES

DATE:__________   WEIGHT:__________   SLEEP:__________   CALORIES:__________

EXERCISES	SETS	REPS	WT	REST	TIME	1 RM	NOTES

DATE:__________   WEIGHT:__________   SLEEP:__________   CALORIES:__________

WORKOUT LOG

NAME:_________________________ GOALS:_________________________

EXERCISES	SETS	REPS	WT	REST	TIME	1 RM	NOTES

DATE:__________ WEIGHT:__________ SLEEP:__________ CALORIES:__________

EXERCISES	SETS	REPS	WT	REST	TIME	1 RM	NOTES

DATE:__________ WEIGHT:__________ SLEEP:__________ CALORIES:__________

EXERCISES	SETS	REPS	WT	REST	TIME	1 RM	NOTES

DATE:__________ WEIGHT:__________ SLEEP:__________ CALORIES:__________

EXERCISES	SETS	REPS	WT	REST	TIME	1 RM	NOTES

DATE:__________ WEIGHT:__________ SLEEP:__________ CALORIES:__________

EXERCISES	SETS	REPS	WT	REST	TIME	1 RM	NOTES

DATE:__________ WEIGHT:__________ SLEEP:__________ CALORIES:__________

WORKOUT LOG

NAME:___________________________   GOALS:___________________________

EXERCISES	SETS	REPS	WT	REST	TIME	1 RM	NOTES

DATE:__________   WEIGHT:__________   SLEEP:__________   CALORIES:__________

EXERCISES	SETS	REPS	WT	REST	TIME	1 RM	NOTES

DATE:__________   WEIGHT:__________   SLEEP:__________   CALORIES:__________

EXERCISES	SETS	REPS	WT	REST	TIME	1 RM	NOTES

DATE:__________   WEIGHT:__________   SLEEP:__________   CALORIES:__________

EXERCISES	SETS	REPS	WT	REST	TIME	1 RM	NOTES

DATE:__________   WEIGHT:__________   SLEEP:__________   CALORIES:__________

EXERCISES	SETS	REPS	WT	REST	TIME	1 RM	NOTES

DATE:__________   WEIGHT:__________   SLEEP:__________   CALORIES:__________

WORKOUT LOG

NAME:_________________________   GOALS:_________________________

EXERCISES	SETS	REPS	WT	REST	TIME	1 RM	NOTES

DATE:_________   WEIGHT:_________   SLEEP:_________   CALORIES:_________

EXERCISES	SETS	REPS	WT	REST	TIME	1 RM	NOTES

DATE:_________   WEIGHT:_________   SLEEP:_________   CALORIES:_________

EXERCISES	SETS	REPS	WT	REST	TIME	1 RM	NOTES

DATE:_________   WEIGHT:_________   SLEEP:_________   CALORIES:_________

EXERCISES	SETS	REPS	WT	REST	TIME	1 RM	NOTES

DATE:_________   WEIGHT:_________   SLEEP:_________   CALORIES:_________

EXERCISES	SETS	REPS	WT	REST	TIME	1 RM	NOTES

DATE:_________   WEIGHT:_________   SLEEP:_________   CALORIES:_________

WORKOUT LOG

NAME:________________________   GOALS:________________________

EXERCISES	SETS	REPS	WT	REST	TIME	1 RM	NOTES

DATE:__________   WEIGHT:__________   SLEEP:__________   CALORIES:__________

EXERCISES	SETS	REPS	WT	REST	TIME	1 RM	NOTES

DATE:__________   WEIGHT:__________   SLEEP:__________   CALORIES:__________

EXERCISES	SETS	REPS	WT	REST	TIME	1 RM	NOTES

DATE:__________   WEIGHT:__________   SLEEP:__________   CALORIES:__________

EXERCISES	SETS	REPS	WT	REST	TIME	1 RM	NOTES

DATE:__________   WEIGHT:__________   SLEEP:__________   CALORIES:__________

EXERCISES	SETS	REPS	WT	REST	TIME	1 RM	NOTES

DATE:__________   WEIGHT:__________   SLEEP:__________   CALORIES:__________

WORKOUT LOG

NAME:___________________________   GOALS:___________________________

EXERCISES	SETS	REPS	WT	REST	TIME	1RM	NOTES

DATE:__________   WEIGHT:__________   SLEEP:__________   CALORIES:__________

EXERCISES	SETS	REPS	WT	REST	TIME	1RM	NOTES

DATE:__________   WEIGHT:__________   SLEEP:__________   CALORIES:__________

EXERCISES	SETS	REPS	WT	REST	TIME	1RM	NOTES

DATE:__________   WEIGHT:__________   SLEEP:__________   CALORIES:__________

EXERCISES	SETS	REPS	WT	REST	TIME	1RM	NOTES

DATE:__________   WEIGHT:__________   SLEEP:__________   CALORIES:__________

EXERCISES	SETS	REPS	WT	REST	TIME	1RM	NOTES

DATE:__________   WEIGHT:__________   SLEEP:__________   CALORIES:__________

WORKOUT LOG

NAME:_________________________ GOALS:_________________________

EXERCISES	SETS	REPS	WT	REST	TIME	1 RM	NOTES

DATE:_________ WEIGHT:_________ SLEEP:_________ CALORIES:_________

EXERCISES	SETS	REPS	WT	REST	TIME	1 RM	NOTES

DATE:_________ WEIGHT:_________ SLEEP:_________ CALORIES:_________

EXERCISES	SETS	REPS	WT	REST	TIME	1 RM	NOTES

DATE:_________ WEIGHT:_________ SLEEP:_________ CALORIES:_________

EXERCISES	SETS	REPS	WT	REST	TIME	1 RM	NOTES

DATE:_________ WEIGHT:_________ SLEEP:_________ CALORIES:_________

EXERCISES	SETS	REPS	WT	REST	TIME	1 RM	NOTES

DATE:_________ WEIGHT:_________ SLEEP:_________ CALORIES:_________

WORKOUT LOG

NAME:________________________   GOALS:__________________________

EXERCISES	SETS	REPS	WT	REST	TIME	1 RM	NOTES

DATE:__________   WEIGHT:__________   SLEEP:__________   CALORIES:__________

EXERCISES	SETS	REPS	WT	REST	TIME	1 RM	NOTES

DATE:__________   WEIGHT:__________   SLEEP:__________   CALORIES:__________

EXERCISES	SETS	REPS	WT	REST	TIME	1 RM	NOTES

DATE:__________   WEIGHT:__________   SLEEP:__________   CALORIES:__________

EXERCISES	SETS	REPS	WT	REST	TIME	1 RM	NOTES

DATE:__________   WEIGHT:__________   SLEEP:__________   CALORIES:__________

EXERCISES	SETS	REPS	WT	REST	TIME	1 RM	NOTES

DATE:__________   WEIGHT:__________   SLEEP:__________   CALORIES:__________

WORKOUT LOG

NAME:_____________________________   GOALS:_____________________________

EXERCISES	SETS	REPS	WT	REST	TIME	1 RM	NOTES

DATE:__________   WEIGHT:__________   SLEEP:__________   CALORIES:__________

EXERCISES	SETS	REPS	WT	REST	TIME	1 RM	NOTES

DATE:__________   WEIGHT:__________   SLEEP:__________   CALORIES:__________

EXERCISES	SETS	REPS	WT	REST	TIME	1 RM	NOTES

DATE:__________   WEIGHT:__________   SLEEP:__________   CALORIES:__________

EXERCISES	SETS	REPS	WT	REST	TIME	1 RM	NOTES

DATE:__________   WEIGHT:__________   SLEEP:__________   CALORIES:__________

EXERCISES	SETS	REPS	WT	REST	TIME	1 RM	NOTES

DATE:__________   WEIGHT:__________   SLEEP:__________   CALORIES:__________

WORKOUT LOG

NAME:________________________ GOALS:____________________

EXERCISES	SETS	REPS	WT	REST	TIME	1 RM	NOTES

DATE:__________   WEIGHT:__________   SLEEP:__________   CALORIES:__________

EXERCISES	SETS	REPS	WT	REST	TIME	1 RM	NOTES

DATE:__________   WEIGHT:__________   SLEEP:__________   CALORIES:__________

EXERCISES	SETS	REPS	WT	REST	TIME	1 RM	NOTES

DATE:__________   WEIGHT:__________   SLEEP:__________   CALORIES:__________

EXERCISES	SETS	REPS	WT	REST	TIME	1 RM	NOTES

DATE:__________   WEIGHT:__________   SLEEP:__________   CALORIES:__________

EXERCISES	SETS	REPS	WT	REST	TIME	1 RM	NOTES

DATE:__________   WEIGHT:__________   SLEEP:__________   CALORIES:__________

WORKOUT LOG

NAME:____________________________   GOALS:____________________________

EXERCISES	SETS	REPS	WT	REST	TIME	1 RM	NOTES

DATE:__________   WEIGHT:__________   SLEEP:__________   CALORIES:__________

EXERCISES	SETS	REPS	WT	REST	TIME	1 RM	NOTES

DATE:__________   WEIGHT:__________   SLEEP:__________   CALORIES:__________

EXERCISES	SETS	REPS	WT	REST	TIME	1 RM	NOTES

DATE:__________   WEIGHT:__________   SLEEP:__________   CALORIES:__________

EXERCISES	SETS	REPS	WT	REST	TIME	1 RM	NOTES

DATE:__________   WEIGHT:__________   SLEEP:__________   CALORIES:__________

EXERCISES	SETS	REPS	WT	REST	TIME	1 RM	NOTES

DATE:__________   WEIGHT:__________   SLEEP:__________   CALORIES:__________

WORKOUT LOG

NAME:______________________ GOALS:____________________

EXERCISES	SETS	REPS	WT	REST	TIME	1 RM	NOTES

DATE:_________   WEIGHT:_________   SLEEP:_________   CALORIES:_________

EXERCISES	SETS	REPS	WT	REST	TIME	1 RM	NOTES

DATE:_________   WEIGHT:_________   SLEEP:_________   CALORIES:_________

EXERCISES	SETS	REPS	WT	REST	TIME	1 RM	NOTES

DATE:_________   WEIGHT:_________   SLEEP:_________   CALORIES:_________

EXERCISES	SETS	REPS	WT	REST	TIME	1 RM	NOTES

DATE:_________   WEIGHT:_________   SLEEP:_________   CALORIES:_________

EXERCISES	SETS	REPS	WT	REST	TIME	1 RM	NOTES

DATE:_________   WEIGHT:_________   SLEEP:_________   CALORIES:_________

WORKOUT LOG

NAME: _________________________   **GOALS:** _________________________

EXERCISES	SETS	REPS	WT	REST	TIME	1 RM	NOTES

DATE: _________   **WEIGHT:** _________   **SLEEP:** _________   **CALORIES:** _________

EXERCISES	SETS	REPS	WT	REST	TIME	1 RM	NOTES

DATE: _________   **WEIGHT:** _________   **SLEEP:** _________   **CALORIES:** _________

EXERCISES	SETS	REPS	WT	REST	TIME	1 RM	NOTES

DATE: _________   **WEIGHT:** _________   **SLEEP:** _________   **CALORIES:** _________

EXERCISES	SETS	REPS	WT	REST	TIME	1 RM	NOTES

DATE: _________   **WEIGHT:** _________   **SLEEP:** _________   **CALORIES:** _________

EXERCISES	SETS	REPS	WT	REST	TIME	1 RM	NOTES

DATE: _________   **WEIGHT:** _________   **SLEEP:** _________   **CALORIES:** _________

WORKOUT LOG

NAME:_________________________   GOALS:___________________________

EXERCISES	SETS	REPS	WT	REST	TIME	1 RM	NOTES

DATE:__________   WEIGHT:__________   SLEEP:__________   CALORIES:__________

EXERCISES	SETS	REPS	WT	REST	TIME	1 RM	NOTES

DATE:__________   WEIGHT:__________   SLEEP:__________   CALORIES:__________

EXERCISES	SETS	REPS	WT	REST	TIME	1 RM	NOTES

DATE:__________   WEIGHT:__________   SLEEP:__________   CALORIES:__________

EXERCISES	SETS	REPS	WT	REST	TIME	1 RM	NOTES

DATE:__________   WEIGHT:__________   SLEEP:__________   CALORIES:__________

EXERCISES	SETS	REPS	WT	REST	TIME	1 RM	NOTES

DATE:__________   WEIGHT:__________   SLEEP:__________   CALORIES:__________

WORKOUT LOG

NAME:________________________ GOALS:________________________

EXERCISES	SETS	REPS	WT	REST	TIME	1 RM	NOTES

DATE:__________ WEIGHT:__________ SLEEP:__________ CALORIES:__________

EXERCISES	SETS	REPS	WT	REST	TIME	1 RM	NOTES

DATE:__________ WEIGHT:__________ SLEEP:__________ CALORIES:__________

EXERCISES	SETS	REPS	WT	REST	TIME	1 RM	NOTES

DATE:__________ WEIGHT:__________ SLEEP:__________ CALORIES:__________

EXERCISES	SETS	REPS	WT	REST	TIME	1 RM	NOTES

DATE:__________ WEIGHT:__________ SLEEP:__________ CALORIES:__________

EXERCISES	SETS	REPS	WT	REST	TIME	1 RM	NOTES

DATE:__________ WEIGHT:__________ SLEEP:__________ CALORIES:__________

WORKOUT LOG

NAME:_____________________________ GOALS:__________________________

EXERCISES	SETS	REPS	WT	REST	TIME	1 RM	NOTES

DATE:_________ WEIGHT:_________ SLEEP:_________ CALORIES:_________

EXERCISES	SETS	REPS	WT	REST	TIME	1 RM	NOTES

DATE:_________ WEIGHT:_________ SLEEP:_________ CALORIES:_________

EXERCISES	SETS	REPS	WT	REST	TIME	1 RM	NOTES

DATE:_________ WEIGHT:_________ SLEEP:_________ CALORIES:_________

EXERCISES	SETS	REPS	WT	REST	TIME	1 RM	NOTES

DATE:_________ WEIGHT:_________ SLEEP:_________ CALORIES:_________

EXERCISES	SETS	REPS	WT	REST	TIME	1 RM	NOTES

DATE:_________ WEIGHT:_________ SLEEP:_________ CALORIES:_________

WORKOUT LOG

NAME:_______________________ GOALS:_______________________

EXERCISES	SETS	REPS	WT	REST	TIME	1 RM	NOTES

DATE:__________ WEIGHT:__________ SLEEP:__________ CALORIES:__________

EXERCISES	SETS	REPS	WT	REST	TIME	1 RM	NOTES

DATE:__________ WEIGHT:__________ SLEEP:__________ CALORIES:__________

EXERCISES	SETS	REPS	WT	REST	TIME	1 RM	NOTES

DATE:__________ WEIGHT:__________ SLEEP:__________ CALORIES:__________

EXERCISES	SETS	REPS	WT	REST	TIME	1 RM	NOTES

DATE:__________ WEIGHT:__________ SLEEP:__________ CALORIES:__________

EXERCISES	SETS	REPS	WT	REST	TIME	1 RM	NOTES

DATE:__________ WEIGHT:__________ SLEEP:__________ CALORIES:__________

WORKOUT LOG

NAME:______________________________ GOALS:______________________________

EXERCISES	SETS	REPS	WT	REST	TIME	1 RM	NOTES

DATE:__________ WEIGHT:__________ SLEEP:__________ CALORIES:__________

EXERCISES	SETS	REPS	WT	REST	TIME	1 RM	NOTES

DATE:__________ WEIGHT:__________ SLEEP:__________ CALORIES:__________

EXERCISES	SETS	REPS	WT	REST	TIME	1 RM	NOTES

DATE:__________ WEIGHT:__________ SLEEP:__________ CALORIES:__________

EXERCISES	SETS	REPS	WT	REST	TIME	1 RM	NOTES

DATE:__________ WEIGHT:__________ SLEEP:__________ CALORIES:__________

EXERCISES	SETS	REPS	WT	REST	TIME	1 RM	NOTES

DATE:__________ WEIGHT:__________ SLEEP:__________ CALORIES:__________

WORKOUT LOG

NAME: _______________________   GOALS: _______________________

EXERCISES	SETS	REPS	WT	REST	TIME	1 RM	NOTES

DATE: _________   WEIGHT: _________   SLEEP: _________   CALORIES: _________

EXERCISES	SETS	REPS	WT	REST	TIME	1 RM	NOTES

DATE: _________   WEIGHT: _________   SLEEP: _________   CALORIES: _________

EXERCISES	SETS	REPS	WT	REST	TIME	1 RM	NOTES

DATE: _________   WEIGHT: _________   SLEEP: _________   CALORIES: _________

EXERCISES	SETS	REPS	WT	REST	TIME	1 RM	NOTES

DATE: _________   WEIGHT: _________   SLEEP: _________   CALORIES: _________

EXERCISES	SETS	REPS	WT	REST	TIME	1 RM	NOTES

DATE: _________   WEIGHT: _________   SLEEP: _________   CALORIES: _________

WORKOUT LOG

NAME:________________________   GOALS:____________________

EXERCISES	SETS	REPS	WT	REST	TIME	1 RM	NOTES

DATE:__________   WEIGHT:__________   SLEEP:__________   CALORIES:__________

EXERCISES	SETS	REPS	WT	REST	TIME	1 RM	NOTES

DATE:__________   WEIGHT:__________   SLEEP:__________   CALORIES:__________

EXERCISES	SETS	REPS	WT	REST	TIME	1 RM	NOTES

DATE:__________   WEIGHT:__________   SLEEP:__________   CALORIES:__________

EXERCISES	SETS	REPS	WT	REST	TIME	1 RM	NOTES

DATE:__________   WEIGHT:__________   SLEEP:__________   CALORIES:__________

EXERCISES	SETS	REPS	WT	REST	TIME	1 RM	NOTES

DATE:__________   WEIGHT:__________   SLEEP:__________   CALORIES:__________

WORKOUT LOG

NAME:________________________   GOALS:____________________

EXERCISES	SETS	REPS	WT	REST	TIME	1RM	NOTES

DATE:__________   WEIGHT:__________   SLEEP:__________   CALORIES:__________

EXERCISES	SETS	REPS	WT	REST	TIME	1RM	NOTES

DATE:__________   WEIGHT:__________   SLEEP:__________   CALORIES:__________

EXERCISES	SETS	REPS	WT	REST	TIME	1RM	NOTES

DATE:__________   WEIGHT:__________   SLEEP:__________   CALORIES:__________

EXERCISES	SETS	REPS	WT	REST	TIME	1RM	NOTES

DATE:__________   WEIGHT:__________   SLEEP:__________   CALORIES:__________

EXERCISES	SETS	REPS	WT	REST	TIME	1RM	NOTES

DATE:__________   WEIGHT:__________   SLEEP:__________   CALORIES:__________

WORKOUT LOG

NAME:_________________________ GOALS:_________________________

EXERCISES	SETS	REPS	WT	REST	TIME	1 RM	NOTES

DATE:__________ WEIGHT:__________ SLEEP:__________ CALORIES:__________

EXERCISES	SETS	REPS	WT	REST	TIME	1 RM	NOTES

DATE:__________ WEIGHT:__________ SLEEP:__________ CALORIES:__________

EXERCISES	SETS	REPS	WT	REST	TIME	1 RM	NOTES

DATE:__________ WEIGHT:__________ SLEEP:__________ CALORIES:__________

EXERCISES	SETS	REPS	WT	REST	TIME	1 RM	NOTES

DATE:__________ WEIGHT:__________ SLEEP:__________ CALORIES:__________

EXERCISES	SETS	REPS	WT	REST	TIME	1 RM	NOTES

DATE:__________ WEIGHT:__________ SLEEP:__________ CALORIES:__________

WORKOUT LOG

NAME:________________________ GOALS:________________________

EXERCISES	SETS	REPS	WT	REST	TIME	1 RM	NOTES

DATE:__________ WEIGHT:__________ SLEEP:__________ CALORIES:__________

EXERCISES	SETS	REPS	WT	REST	TIME	1 RM	NOTES

DATE:__________ WEIGHT:__________ SLEEP:__________ CALORIES:__________

EXERCISES	SETS	REPS	WT	REST	TIME	1 RM	NOTES

DATE:__________ WEIGHT:__________ SLEEP:__________ CALORIES:__________

EXERCISES	SETS	REPS	WT	REST	TIME	1 RM	NOTES

DATE:__________ WEIGHT:__________ SLEEP:__________ CALORIES:__________

EXERCISES	SETS	REPS	WT	REST	TIME	1 RM	NOTES

DATE:__________ WEIGHT:__________ SLEEP:__________ CALORIES:__________

WORKOUT LOG

NAME:_________________________   GOALS:_________________________

EXERCISES	SETS	REPS	WT	REST	TIME	1 RM	NOTES

DATE:__________   WEIGHT:__________   SLEEP:__________   CALORIES:__________

EXERCISES	SETS	REPS	WT	REST	TIME	1 RM	NOTES

DATE:__________   WEIGHT:__________   SLEEP:__________   CALORIES:__________

EXERCISES	SETS	REPS	WT	REST	TIME	1 RM	NOTES

DATE:__________   WEIGHT:__________   SLEEP:__________   CALORIES:__________

EXERCISES	SETS	REPS	WT	REST	TIME	1 RM	NOTES

DATE:__________   WEIGHT:__________   SLEEP:__________   CALORIES:__________

EXERCISES	SETS	REPS	WT	REST	TIME	1 RM	NOTES

DATE:__________   WEIGHT:__________   SLEEP:__________   CALORIES:__________

WORKOUT LOG

NAME:______________________________   GOALS:______________________________

EXERCISES	SETS	REPS	WT	REST	TIME	1 RM	NOTES

DATE:__________   WEIGHT:__________   SLEEP:__________   CALORIES:__________

EXERCISES	SETS	REPS	WT	REST	TIME	1 RM	NOTES

DATE:__________   WEIGHT:__________   SLEEP:__________   CALORIES:__________

EXERCISES	SETS	REPS	WT	REST	TIME	1 RM	NOTES

DATE:__________   WEIGHT:__________   SLEEP:__________   CALORIES:__________

EXERCISES	SETS	REPS	WT	REST	TIME	1 RM	NOTES

DATE:__________   WEIGHT:__________   SLEEP:__________   CALORIES:__________

EXERCISES	SETS	REPS	WT	REST	TIME	1 RM	NOTES

DATE:__________   WEIGHT:__________   SLEEP:__________   CALORIES:__________

WORKOUT LOG

NAME:__________________________ GOALS:____________________________

EXERCISES	SETS	REPS	WT	REST	TIME	1 RM	NOTES

DATE:__________ WEIGHT:__________ SLEEP:__________ CALORIES:__________

EXERCISES	SETS	REPS	WT	REST	TIME	1 RM	NOTES

DATE:__________ WEIGHT:__________ SLEEP:__________ CALORIES:__________

EXERCISES	SETS	REPS	WT	REST	TIME	1 RM	NOTES

DATE:__________ WEIGHT:__________ SLEEP:__________ CALORIES:__________

EXERCISES	SETS	REPS	WT	REST	TIME	1 RM	NOTES

DATE:__________ WEIGHT:__________ SLEEP:__________ CALORIES:__________

EXERCISES	SETS	REPS	WT	REST	TIME	1 RM	NOTES

DATE:__________ WEIGHT:__________ SLEEP:__________ CALORIES:__________

WORKOUT LOG

NAME:___________________________ GOALS:___________________________

EXERCISES	SETS	REPS	WT	REST	TIME	1 RM	NOTES

DATE:__________   WEIGHT:__________   SLEEP:__________   CALORIES:__________

EXERCISES	SETS	REPS	WT	REST	TIME	1 RM	NOTES

DATE:__________   WEIGHT:__________   SLEEP:__________   CALORIES:__________

EXERCISES	SETS	REPS	WT	REST	TIME	1 RM	NOTES

DATE:__________   WEIGHT:__________   SLEEP:__________   CALORIES:__________

EXERCISES	SETS	REPS	WT	REST	TIME	1 RM	NOTES

DATE:__________   WEIGHT:__________   SLEEP:__________   CALORIES:__________

EXERCISES	SETS	REPS	WT	REST	TIME	1 RM	NOTES

DATE:__________   WEIGHT:__________   SLEEP:__________   CALORIES:__________

WORKOUT LOG

NAME:__________________________ GOALS:__________________________

EXERCISES	SETS	REPS	WT	REST	TIME	1 RM	NOTES

DATE:__________ WEIGHT:__________ SLEEP:__________ CALORIES:__________

EXERCISES	SETS	REPS	WT	REST	TIME	1 RM	NOTES

DATE:__________ WEIGHT:__________ SLEEP:__________ CALORIES:__________

EXERCISES	SETS	REPS	WT	REST	TIME	1 RM	NOTES

DATE:__________ WEIGHT:__________ SLEEP:__________ CALORIES:__________

EXERCISES	SETS	REPS	WT	REST	TIME	1 RM	NOTES

DATE:__________ WEIGHT:__________ SLEEP:__________ CALORIES:__________

EXERCISES	SETS	REPS	WT	REST	TIME	1 RM	NOTES

DATE:__________ WEIGHT:__________ SLEEP:__________ CALORIES:__________

WORKOUT LOG

NAME:_____________________________ GOALS:_____________________________

EXERCISES	SETS	REPS	WT	REST	TIME	1 RM	NOTES

DATE:__________   WEIGHT:__________   SLEEP:__________   CALORIES:__________

EXERCISES	SETS	REPS	WT	REST	TIME	1 RM	NOTES

DATE:__________   WEIGHT:__________   SLEEP:__________   CALORIES:__________

EXERCISES	SETS	REPS	WT	REST	TIME	1 RM	NOTES

DATE:__________   WEIGHT:__________   SLEEP:__________   CALORIES:__________

EXERCISES	SETS	REPS	WT	REST	TIME	1 RM	NOTES

DATE:__________   WEIGHT:__________   SLEEP:__________   CALORIES:__________

EXERCISES	SETS	REPS	WT	REST	TIME	1 RM	NOTES

DATE:__________   WEIGHT:__________   SLEEP:__________   CALORIES:__________

WORKOUT LOG

NAME:_________________________ GOALS:_____________________

EXERCISES	SETS	REPS	WT	REST	TIME	1 RM	NOTES

DATE:___________ WEIGHT:___________ SLEEP:___________ CALORIES:___________

EXERCISES	SETS	REPS	WT	REST	TIME	1 RM	NOTES

DATE:___________ WEIGHT:___________ SLEEP:___________ CALORIES:___________

EXERCISES	SETS	REPS	WT	REST	TIME	1 RM	NOTES

DATE:___________ WEIGHT:___________ SLEEP:___________ CALORIES:___________

EXERCISES	SETS	REPS	WT	REST	TIME	1 RM	NOTES

DATE:___________ WEIGHT:___________ SLEEP:___________ CALORIES:___________

EXERCISES	SETS	REPS	WT	REST	TIME	1 RM	NOTES

DATE:___________ WEIGHT:___________ SLEEP:___________ CALORIES:___________

WORKOUT LOG

NAME:______________________   GOALS:______________________

EXERCISES	SETS	REPS	WT	REST	TIME	1 RM	NOTES

DATE:__________   WEIGHT:__________   SLEEP:__________   CALORIES:__________

EXERCISES	SETS	REPS	WT	REST	TIME	1 RM	NOTES

DATE:__________   WEIGHT:__________   SLEEP:__________   CALORIES:__________

EXERCISES	SETS	REPS	WT	REST	TIME	1 RM	NOTES

DATE:__________   WEIGHT:__________   SLEEP:__________   CALORIES:__________

EXERCISES	SETS	REPS	WT	REST	TIME	1 RM	NOTES

DATE:__________   WEIGHT:__________   SLEEP:__________   CALORIES:__________

EXERCISES	SETS	REPS	WT	REST	TIME	1 RM	NOTES

DATE:__________   WEIGHT:__________   SLEEP:__________   CALORIES:__________

WORKOUT LOG

NAME:_________________________   GOALS:_________________________

EXERCISES	SETS	REPS	WT	REST	TIME	1RM	NOTES

DATE:_________   WEIGHT:_________   SLEEP:_________   CALORIES:_________

EXERCISES	SETS	REPS	WT	REST	TIME	1RM	NOTES

DATE:_________   WEIGHT:_________   SLEEP:_________   CALORIES:_________

EXERCISES	SETS	REPS	WT	REST	TIME	1RM	NOTES

DATE:_________   WEIGHT:_________   SLEEP:_________   CALORIES:_________

EXERCISES	SETS	REPS	WT	REST	TIME	1RM	NOTES

DATE:_________   WEIGHT:_________   SLEEP:_________   CALORIES:_________

EXERCISES	SETS	REPS	WT	REST	TIME	1RM	NOTES

DATE:_________   WEIGHT:_________   SLEEP:_________   CALORIES:_________

WORKOUT LOG

NAME:________________________ GOALS:________________________

EXERCISES	SETS	REPS	WT	REST	TIME	1 RM	NOTES

DATE:__________   WEIGHT:__________   SLEEP:__________   CALORIES:__________

EXERCISES	SETS	REPS	WT	REST	TIME	1 RM	NOTES

DATE:__________   WEIGHT:__________   SLEEP:__________   CALORIES:__________

EXERCISES	SETS	REPS	WT	REST	TIME	1 RM	NOTES

DATE:__________   WEIGHT:__________   SLEEP:__________   CALORIES:__________

EXERCISES	SETS	REPS	WT	REST	TIME	1 RM	NOTES

DATE:__________   WEIGHT:__________   SLEEP:__________   CALORIES:__________

EXERCISES	SETS	REPS	WT	REST	TIME	1 RM	NOTES

DATE:__________   WEIGHT:__________   SLEEP:__________   CALORIES:__________

WORKOUT LOG

NAME:_________________________   GOALS:___________________________

EXERCISES	SETS	REPS	WT	REST	TIME	1 RM	NOTES

DATE:_________   WEIGHT:_________   SLEEP:_________   CALORIES:_________

EXERCISES	SETS	REPS	WT	REST	TIME	1 RM	NOTES

DATE:_________   WEIGHT:_________   SLEEP:_________   CALORIES:_________

EXERCISES	SETS	REPS	WT	REST	TIME	1 RM	NOTES

DATE:_________   WEIGHT:_________   SLEEP:_________   CALORIES:_________

EXERCISES	SETS	REPS	WT	REST	TIME	1 RM	NOTES

DATE:_________   WEIGHT:_________   SLEEP:_________   CALORIES:_________

EXERCISES	SETS	REPS	WT	REST	TIME	1 RM	NOTES

DATE:_________   WEIGHT:_________   SLEEP:_________   CALORIES:_________

WORKOUT LOG

NAME:____________________________ GOALS:____________________________

EXERCISES	SETS	REPS	WT	REST	TIME	1 RM	NOTES

DATE:__________ WEIGHT:__________ SLEEP:__________ CALORIES:__________

EXERCISES	SETS	REPS	WT	REST	TIME	1 RM	NOTES

DATE:__________ WEIGHT:__________ SLEEP:__________ CALORIES:__________

EXERCISES	SETS	REPS	WT	REST	TIME	1 RM	NOTES

DATE:__________ WEIGHT:__________ SLEEP:__________ CALORIES:__________

EXERCISES	SETS	REPS	WT	REST	TIME	1 RM	NOTES

DATE:__________ WEIGHT:__________ SLEEP:__________ CALORIES:__________

EXERCISES	SETS	REPS	WT	REST	TIME	1 RM	NOTES

DATE:__________ WEIGHT:__________ SLEEP:__________ CALORIES:__________

WORKOUT LOG

NAME:_____________________ GOALS:_____________________

EXERCISES	SETS	REPS	WT	REST	TIME	1 RM	NOTES

DATE:_________ WEIGHT:_________ SLEEP:_________ CALORIES:_________

EXERCISES	SETS	REPS	WT	REST	TIME	1 RM	NOTES

DATE:_________ WEIGHT:_________ SLEEP:_________ CALORIES:_________

EXERCISES	SETS	REPS	WT	REST	TIME	1 RM	NOTES

DATE:_________ WEIGHT:_________ SLEEP:_________ CALORIES:_________

EXERCISES	SETS	REPS	WT	REST	TIME	1 RM	NOTES

DATE:_________ WEIGHT:_________ SLEEP:_________ CALORIES:_________

EXERCISES	SETS	REPS	WT	REST	TIME	1 RM	NOTES

DATE:_________ WEIGHT:_________ SLEEP:_________ CALORIES:_________

WORKOUT LOG

NAME:________________________ GOALS:__________________________

EXERCISES	SETS	REPS	WT	REST	TIME	1RM	NOTES

DATE:__________ WEIGHT:__________ SLEEP:__________ CALORIES:__________

EXERCISES	SETS	REPS	WT	REST	TIME	1RM	NOTES

DATE:__________ WEIGHT:__________ SLEEP:__________ CALORIES:__________

EXERCISES	SETS	REPS	WT	REST	TIME	1RM	NOTES

DATE:__________ WEIGHT:__________ SLEEP:__________ CALORIES:__________

EXERCISES	SETS	REPS	WT	REST	TIME	1RM	NOTES

DATE:__________ WEIGHT:__________ SLEEP:__________ CALORIES:__________

EXERCISES	SETS	REPS	WT	REST	TIME	1RM	NOTES

DATE:__________ WEIGHT:__________ SLEEP:__________ CALORIES:__________

WORKOUT LOG

NAME:_________________________ GOALS:_________________________

EXERCISES	SETS	REPS	WT	REST	TIME	1 RM	NOTES

DATE:__________   WEIGHT:__________   SLEEP:__________   CALORIES:__________

EXERCISES	SETS	REPS	WT	REST	TIME	1 RM	NOTES

DATE:__________   WEIGHT:__________   SLEEP:__________   CALORIES:__________

EXERCISES	SETS	REPS	WT	REST	TIME	1 RM	NOTES

DATE:__________   WEIGHT:__________   SLEEP:__________   CALORIES:__________

EXERCISES	SETS	REPS	WT	REST	TIME	1 RM	NOTES

DATE:__________   WEIGHT:__________   SLEEP:__________   CALORIES:__________

EXERCISES	SETS	REPS	WT	REST	TIME	1 RM	NOTES

DATE:__________   WEIGHT:__________   SLEEP:__________   CALORIES:__________

WORKOUT LOG

NAME:__________________________ GOALS:__________________________

EXERCISES	SETS	REPS	WT	REST	TIME	1 RM	NOTES

DATE:__________ WEIGHT:__________ SLEEP:__________ CALORIES:__________

EXERCISES	SETS	REPS	WT	REST	TIME	1 RM	NOTES

DATE:__________ WEIGHT:__________ SLEEP:__________ CALORIES:__________

EXERCISES	SETS	REPS	WT	REST	TIME	1 RM	NOTES

DATE:__________ WEIGHT:__________ SLEEP:__________ CALORIES:__________

EXERCISES	SETS	REPS	WT	REST	TIME	1 RM	NOTES

DATE:__________ WEIGHT:__________ SLEEP:__________ CALORIES:__________

EXERCISES	SETS	REPS	WT	REST	TIME	1 RM	NOTES

DATE:__________ WEIGHT:__________ SLEEP:__________ CALORIES:__________

WORKOUT LOG

NAME:_______________________ GOALS:_______________________

EXERCISES	SETS	REPS	WT	REST	TIME	1 RM	NOTES

DATE:__________ WEIGHT:__________ SLEEP:__________ CALORIES:__________

EXERCISES	SETS	REPS	WT	REST	TIME	1 RM	NOTES

DATE:__________ WEIGHT:__________ SLEEP:__________ CALORIES:__________

EXERCISES	SETS	REPS	WT	REST	TIME	1 RM	NOTES

DATE:__________ WEIGHT:__________ SLEEP:__________ CALORIES:__________

EXERCISES	SETS	REPS	WT	REST	TIME	1 RM	NOTES

DATE:__________ WEIGHT:__________ SLEEP:__________ CALORIES:__________

EXERCISES	SETS	REPS	WT	REST	TIME	1 RM	NOTES

DATE:__________ WEIGHT:__________ SLEEP:__________ CALORIES:__________

WORKOUT LOG

NAME:___________________________   GOALS:___________________________

EXERCISES	SETS	REPS	WT	REST	TIME	1 RM	NOTES

DATE:__________   WEIGHT:__________   SLEEP:__________   CALORIES:__________

EXERCISES	SETS	REPS	WT	REST	TIME	1 RM	NOTES

DATE:__________   WEIGHT:__________   SLEEP:__________   CALORIES:__________

EXERCISES	SETS	REPS	WT	REST	TIME	1 RM	NOTES

DATE:__________   WEIGHT:__________   SLEEP:__________   CALORIES:__________

EXERCISES	SETS	REPS	WT	REST	TIME	1 RM	NOTES

DATE:__________   WEIGHT:__________   SLEEP:__________   CALORIES:__________

EXERCISES	SETS	REPS	WT	REST	TIME	1 RM	NOTES

DATE:__________   WEIGHT:__________   SLEEP:__________   CALORIES:__________

WORKOUT LOG

NAME:_________________________   GOALS:___________________________

EXERCISES	SETS	REPS	WT	REST	TIME	1 RM	NOTES

DATE:___________   WEIGHT:___________   SLEEP:___________   CALORIES:___________

EXERCISES	SETS	REPS	WT	REST	TIME	1 RM	NOTES

DATE:___________   WEIGHT:___________   SLEEP:___________   CALORIES:___________

EXERCISES	SETS	REPS	WT	REST	TIME	1 RM	NOTES

DATE:___________   WEIGHT:___________   SLEEP:___________   CALORIES:___________

EXERCISES	SETS	REPS	WT	REST	TIME	1 RM	NOTES

DATE:___________   WEIGHT:___________   SLEEP:___________   CALORIES:___________

EXERCISES	SETS	REPS	WT	REST	TIME	1 RM	NOTES

DATE:___________   WEIGHT:___________   SLEEP:___________   CALORIES:___________

WORKOUT LOG

NAME:_______________________ GOALS:_______________________

EXERCISES	SETS	REPS	WT	REST	TIME	1 RM	NOTES

DATE:__________ WEIGHT:__________ SLEEP:__________ CALORIES:__________

EXERCISES	SETS	REPS	WT	REST	TIME	1 RM	NOTES

DATE:__________ WEIGHT:__________ SLEEP:__________ CALORIES:__________

EXERCISES	SETS	REPS	WT	REST	TIME	1 RM	NOTES

DATE:__________ WEIGHT:__________ SLEEP:__________ CALORIES:__________

EXERCISES	SETS	REPS	WT	REST	TIME	1 RM	NOTES

DATE:__________ WEIGHT:__________ SLEEP:__________ CALORIES:__________

EXERCISES	SETS	REPS	WT	REST	TIME	1 RM	NOTES

DATE:__________ WEIGHT:__________ SLEEP:__________ CALORIES:__________

WORKOUT LOG

NAME:___________________________ GOALS:___________________________

EXERCISES	SETS	REPS	WT	REST	TIME	1 RM	NOTES

DATE:___________ WEIGHT:___________ SLEEP:___________ CALORIES:___________

EXERCISES	SETS	REPS	WT	REST	TIME	1 RM	NOTES

DATE:___________ WEIGHT:___________ SLEEP:___________ CALORIES:___________

EXERCISES	SETS	REPS	WT	REST	TIME	1 RM	NOTES

DATE:___________ WEIGHT:___________ SLEEP:___________ CALORIES:___________

EXERCISES	SETS	REPS	WT	REST	TIME	1 RM	NOTES

DATE:___________ WEIGHT:___________ SLEEP:___________ CALORIES:___________

EXERCISES	SETS	REPS	WT	REST	TIME	1 RM	NOTES

DATE:___________ WEIGHT:___________ SLEEP:___________ CALORIES:___________

WORKOUT LOG

NAME:__________________________   GOALS:__________________________

EXERCISES	SETS	REPS	WT	REST	TIME	1 RM	NOTES

DATE:__________   WEIGHT:__________   SLEEP:__________   CALORIES:__________

EXERCISES	SETS	REPS	WT	REST	TIME	1 RM	NOTES

DATE:__________   WEIGHT:__________   SLEEP:__________   CALORIES:__________

EXERCISES	SETS	REPS	WT	REST	TIME	1 RM	NOTES

DATE:__________   WEIGHT:__________   SLEEP:__________   CALORIES:__________

EXERCISES	SETS	REPS	WT	REST	TIME	1 RM	NOTES

DATE:__________   WEIGHT:__________   SLEEP:__________   CALORIES:__________

EXERCISES	SETS	REPS	WT	REST	TIME	1 RM	NOTES

DATE:__________   WEIGHT:__________   SLEEP:__________   CALORIES:__________

WORKOUT LOG

NAME:____________________________ GOALS:____________________________

EXERCISES	SETS	REPS	WT	REST	TIME	1 RM	NOTES

DATE:__________ WEIGHT:__________ SLEEP:__________ CALORIES:__________

EXERCISES	SETS	REPS	WT	REST	TIME	1 RM	NOTES

DATE:__________ WEIGHT:__________ SLEEP:__________ CALORIES:__________

EXERCISES	SETS	REPS	WT	REST	TIME	1 RM	NOTES

DATE:__________ WEIGHT:__________ SLEEP:__________ CALORIES:__________

EXERCISES	SETS	REPS	WT	REST	TIME	1 RM	NOTES

DATE:__________ WEIGHT:__________ SLEEP:__________ CALORIES:__________

EXERCISES	SETS	REPS	WT	REST	TIME	1 RM	NOTES

DATE:__________ WEIGHT:__________ SLEEP:__________ CALORIES:__________

WORKOUT LOG

NAME:_________________________ GOALS:_________________________

EXERCISES	SETS	REPS	WT	REST	TIME	1 RM	NOTES

DATE:_________ WEIGHT:_________ SLEEP:_________ CALORIES:_________

EXERCISES	SETS	REPS	WT	REST	TIME	1 RM	NOTES

DATE:_________ WEIGHT:_________ SLEEP:_________ CALORIES:_________

EXERCISES	SETS	REPS	WT	REST	TIME	1 RM	NOTES

DATE:_________ WEIGHT:_________ SLEEP:_________ CALORIES:_________

EXERCISES	SETS	REPS	WT	REST	TIME	1 RM	NOTES

DATE:_________ WEIGHT:_________ SLEEP:_________ CALORIES:_________

EXERCISES	SETS	REPS	WT	REST	TIME	1 RM	NOTES

DATE:_________ WEIGHT:_________ SLEEP:_________ CALORIES:_________

WORKOUT LOG

NAME: _____________________________   GOALS: _____________________________

EXERCISES	SETS	REPS	WT	REST	TIME	1 RM	NOTES

DATE: __________   WEIGHT: __________   SLEEP: __________   CALORIES: __________

EXERCISES	SETS	REPS	WT	REST	TIME	1 RM	NOTES

DATE: __________   WEIGHT: __________   SLEEP: __________   CALORIES: __________

EXCROISES	SETS	REPS	WT	REST	TIME	1 RM	NOTES

DATE: __________   WEIGHT: __________   SLEEP: __________   CALORIES: __________

EXERCISES	SETS	REPS	WT	REST	TIME	1 RM	NOTES

DATE: __________   WEIGHT: __________   SLEEP: __________   CALORIES: __________

EXERCISES	SETS	REPS	WT	REST	TIME	1 RM	NOTES

DATE: __________   WEIGHT: __________   SLEEP: __________   CALORIES: __________

WORKOUT LOG

NAME:________________________ GOALS:________________________

EXERCISES	SETS	REPS	WT	REST	TIME	1 RM	NOTES

DATE:__________ WEIGHT:__________ SLEEP:__________ CALORIES:__________

EXERCISES	SETS	REPS	WT	REST	TIME	1 RM	NOTES

DATE:__________ WEIGHT:__________ SLEEP:__________ CALORIES:__________

EXERCISES	SETS	REPS	WT	REST	TIME	1 RM	NOTES

DATE:__________ WEIGHT:__________ SLEEP:__________ CALORIES:__________

EXERCISES	SETS	REPS	WT	REST	TIME	1 RM	NOTES

DATE:__________ WEIGHT:__________ SLEEP:__________ CALORIES:__________

EXERCISES	SETS	REPS	WT	REST	TIME	1 RM	NOTES

DATE:__________ WEIGHT:__________ SLEEP:__________ CALORIES:__________

WORKOUT LOG

NAME:________________________   GOALS:__________________________

EXERCISES	SETS	REPS	WT	REST	TIME	1 RM	NOTES

DATE:__________   WEIGHT:__________   SLEEP:__________   CALORIES:__________

EXERCISES	SETS	REPS	WT	REST	TIME	1 RM	NOTES

DATE:__________   WEIGHT:__________   SLEEP:__________   CALORIES:__________

EXERCISES	SETS	REPS	WT	REST	TIME	1 RM	NOTES

DATE:__________   WEIGHT:__________   SLEEP:__________   CALORIES:__________

EXERCISES	SETS	REPS	WT	REST	TIME	1 RM	NOTES

DATE:__________   WEIGHT:__________   SLEEP:__________   CALORIES:__________

EXERCISES	SETS	REPS	WT	REST	TIME	1 RM	NOTES

DATE:__________   WEIGHT:__________   SLEEP:__________   CALORIES:__________

WORKOUT LOG

NAME:_________________________   GOALS:_____________________

EXERCISES	SETS	REPS	WT	REST	TIME	1 RM	NOTES

DATE:_________   WEIGHT:_________   SLEEP:_________   CALORIES:_________

EXERCISES	SETS	REPS	WT	REST	TIME	1 RM	NOTES

DATE:_________   WEIGHT:_________   SLEEP:_________   CALORIES:_________

EXERCISES	SETS	REPS	WT	REST	TIME	1 RM	NOTES

DATE:_________   WEIGHT:_________   SLEEP:_________   CALORIES:_________

EXERCISES	SETS	REPS	WT	REST	TIME	1 RM	NOTES

DATE:_________   WEIGHT:_________   SLEEP:_________   CALORIES:_________

EXERCISES	SETS	REPS	WT	REST	TIME	1 RM	NOTES

DATE:_________   WEIGHT:_________   SLEEP:_________   CALORIES:_________

WORKOUT LOG

NAME:_____________________________   GOALS:_____________________________

EXERCISES	SETS	REPS	WT	REST	TIME	1 RM	NOTES

DATE:__________   WEIGHT:__________   SLEEP:__________   CALORIES:__________

EXERCISES	SETS	REPS	WT	REST	TIME	1 RM	NOTES

DATE:__________   WEIGHT:__________   SLEEP:__________   CALORIES:__________

EXERCISES	SETS	REPS	WT	REST	TIME	1 RM	NOTES

DATE:__________   WEIGHT:__________   SLEEP:__________   CALORIES:__________

EXERCISES	SETS	REPS	WT	REST	TIME	1 RM	NOTES

DATE:__________   WEIGHT:__________   SLEEP:__________   CALORIES:__________

EXERCISES	SETS	REPS	WT	REST	TIME	1 RM	NOTES

DATE:__________   WEIGHT:__________   SLEEP:__________   CALORIES:__________

WORKOUT LOG

NAME:_____________________ GOALS:_____________________

EXERCISES	SETS	REPS	WT	REST	TIME	1RM	NOTES

DATE:__________ WEIGHT:__________ SLEEP:__________ CALORIES:__________

EXERCISES	SETS	REPS	WT	REST	TIME	1RM	NOTES

DATE:__________ WEIGHT:__________ SLEEP:__________ CALORIES:__________

EXERCISES	SETS	REPS	WT	REST	TIME	1RM	NOTES

DATE:__________ WEIGHT:__________ SLEEP:__________ CALORIES:__________

EXERCISES	SETS	REPS	WT	REST	TIME	1RM	NOTES

DATE:__________ WEIGHT:__________ SLEEP:__________ CALORIES:__________

EXERCISES	SETS	REPS	WT	REST	TIME	1RM	NOTES

DATE:__________ WEIGHT:__________ SLEEP:__________ CALORIES:__________

WORKOUT LOG

NAME:________________________   GOALS:________________________

EXERCISES	SETS	REPS	WT	REST	TIME	1 RM	NOTES

DATE:__________   WEIGHT:__________   SLEEP:__________   CALORIES:__________

EXERCISES	SETS	REPS	WT	REST	TIME	1 RM	NOTES

DATE:__________   WEIGHT:__________   SLEEP:__________   CALORIES:__________

EXERCISES	SETS	REPS	WT	REST	TIME	1 RM	NOTES

DATE:__________   WEIGHT:__________   SLEEP:__________   CALORIES:__________

EXERCISES	SETS	REPS	WT	REST	TIME	1 RM	NOTES

DATE:__________   WEIGHT:__________   SLEEP:__________   CALORIES:__________

EXERCISES	SETS	REPS	WT	REST	TIME	1 RM	NOTES

DATE:__________   WEIGHT:__________   SLEEP:__________   CALORIES:__________

WORKOUT LOG

NAME:_________________________   GOALS:_________________________

EXERCISES	SETS	REPS	WT	REST	TIME	1 RM	NOTES

DATE:_________   WEIGHT:_________   SLEEP:_________   CALORIES:_________

EXERCISES	SETS	REPS	WT	REST	TIME	1 RM	NOTES

DATE:_________   WEIGHT:_________   SLEEP:_________   CALORIES:_________

EXERCISES	SETS	REPS	WT	REST	TIME	1 RM	NOTES

DATE:_________   WEIGHT:_________   SLEEP:_________   CALORIES:_________

EXERCISES	SETS	REPS	WT	REST	TIME	1 RM	NOTES

DATE:_________   WEIGHT:_________   SLEEP:_________   CALORIES:_________

EXERCISES	SETS	REPS	WT	REST	TIME	1 RM	NOTES

DATE:_________   WEIGHT:_________   SLEEP:_________   CALORIES:_________

WORKOUT LOG

NAME:_____________________   GOALS:_____________________

EXERCISES	SETS	REPS	WT	REST	TIME	1 RM	NOTES

DATE:_________   WEIGHT:_________   SLEEP:_________   CALORIES:_________

EXERCISES	SETS	REPS	WT	REST	TIME	1 RM	NOTES

DATE:_________   WEIGHT:_________   SLEEP:_________   CALORIES:_________

EXERCISES	SETS	REPS	WT	REST	TIME	1 RM	NOTES

DATE:_________   WEIGHT:_________   SLEEP:_________   CALORIES:_________

EXERCISES	SETS	REPS	WT	REST	TIME	1 RM	NOTES

DATE:_________   WEIGHT:_________   SLEEP:_________   CALORIES:_________

EXERCISES	SETS	REPS	WT	REST	TIME	1 RM	NOTES

DATE:_________   WEIGHT:_________   SLEEP:_________   CALORIES:_________

WORKOUT LOG

NAME:__________________________ GOALS:__________________________

EXERCISES	SETS	REPS	WT	REST	TIME	1 RM	NOTES

DATE:__________ WEIGHT:__________ SLEEP:__________ CALORIES:__________

EXERCISES	SETS	REPS	WT	REST	TIME	1 RM	NOTES

DATE:__________ WEIGHT:__________ SLEEP:__________ CALORIES:__________

EXERCISES	SETS	REPS	WT	REST	TIME	1 RM	NOTES

DATE:__________ WEIGHT:__________ SLEEP:__________ CALORIES:__________

EXERCISES	SETS	REPS	WT	REST	TIME	1 RM	NOTES

DATE:__________ WEIGHT:__________ SLEEP:__________ CALORIES:__________

EXERCISES	SETS	REPS	WT	REST	TIME	1 RM	NOTES

DATE:__________ WEIGHT:__________ SLEEP:__________ CALORIES:__________

WORKOUT LOG

NAME:_________________________ GOALS:_________________________

EXERCISES	SETS	REPS	WT	REST	TIME	1 RM	NOTES

DATE:_________ WEIGHT:_________ SLEEP:_________ CALORIES:_________

EXERCISES	SETS	REPS	WT	REST	TIME	1 RM	NOTES

DATE:_________ WEIGHT:_________ SLEEP:_________ CALORIES:_________

EXERCISES	SETS	REPS	WT	REST	TIME	1 RM	NOTES

DATE:_________ WEIGHT:_________ SLEEP:_________ CALORIES:_________

EXERCISES	SETS	REPS	WT	REST	TIME	1 RM	NOTES

DATE:_________ WEIGHT:_________ SLEEP:_________ CALORIES:_________

EXERCISES	SETS	REPS	WT	REST	TIME	1 RM	NOTES

DATE:_________ WEIGHT:_________ SLEEP:_________ CALORIES:_________

WORKOUT LOG

NAME:______________________ GOALS:______________________

EXERCISES	SETS	REPS	WT	REST	TIME	1 RM	NOTES

DATE:__________ WEIGHT:__________ SLEEP:__________ CALORIES:__________

EXERCISES	SETS	REPS	WT	REST	TIME	1 RM	NOTES

DATE:__________ WEIGHT:__________ SLEEP:__________ CALORIES:__________

EXERCISES	SETS	REPS	WT	REST	TIME	1 RM	NOTES

DATE:__________ WEIGHT:__________ SLEEP:__________ CALORIES:__________

EXERCISES	SETS	REPS	WT	REST	TIME	1 RM	NOTES

DATE:__________ WEIGHT:__________ SLEEP:__________ CALORIES:__________

EXERCISES	SETS	REPS	WT	REST	TIME	1 RM	NOTES

DATE:__________ WEIGHT:__________ SLEEP:__________ CALORIES:__________

WORKOUT LOG

NAME:_____________________________   GOALS:_____________________________

EXERCISES	SETS	REPS	WT	REST	TIME	1 RM	NOTES

DATE:__________   WEIGHT:__________   SLEEP:__________   CALORIES:__________

EXERCISES	SETS	REPS	WT	REST	TIME	1 RM	NOTES

DATE:__________   WEIGHT:__________   SLEEP:__________   CALORIES:__________

EXERCISES	SETS	REPS	WT	REST	TIME	1 RM	NOTES

DATE:__________   WEIGHT:__________   SLEEP:__________   CALORIES:__________

EXERCISES	SETS	REPS	WT	REST	TIME	1 RM	NOTES

DATE:__________   WEIGHT:__________   SLEEP:__________   CALORIES:__________

EXERCISES	SETS	REPS	WT	REST	TIME	1 RM	NOTES

DATE:__________   WEIGHT:__________   SLEEP:__________   CALORIES:__________

WORKOUT LOG

NAME: _______________________ GOALS: _______________________

EXERCISES	SETS	REPS	WT	REST	TIME	1 RM	NOTES

DATE: __________ WEIGHT: __________ SLEEP: __________ CALORIES: __________

EXERCISES	SETS	REPS	WT	REST	TIME	1 RM	NOTES

DATE: __________ WEIGHT: __________ SLEEP: __________ CALORIES: __________

EXERCISES	SETS	REPS	WT	REST	TIME	1 RM	NOTES

DATE: __________ WEIGHT: __________ SLEEP: __________ CALORIES: __________

EXERCISES	SETS	REPS	WT	REST	TIME	1 RM	NOTES

DATE: __________ WEIGHT: __________ SLEEP: __________ CALORIES: __________

EXERCISES	SETS	REPS	WT	REST	TIME	1 RM	NOTES

DATE: __________ WEIGHT: __________ SLEEP: __________ CALORIES: __________

WORKOUT LOG

NAME:_________________________ GOALS:_____________________

EXERCISES	SETS	REPS	WT	REST	TIME	1 RM	NOTES

DATE:__________ WEIGHT:__________ SLEEP:__________ CALORIES:__________

EXERCISES	SETS	REPS	WT	REST	TIME	1 RM	NOTES

DATE:__________ WEIGHT:__________ SLEEP:__________ CALORIES:__________

EXERCISES	SETS	REPS	WT	REST	TIME	1 RM	NOTES

DATE:__________ WEIGHT:__________ SLEEP:__________ CALORIES:__________

EXERCISES	SETS	REPS	WT	REST	TIME	1 RM	NOTES

DATE:__________ WEIGHT:__________ SLEEP:__________ CALORIES:__________

EXERCISES	SETS	REPS	WT	REST	TIME	1 RM	NOTES

DATE:__________ WEIGHT:__________ SLEEP:__________ CALORIES:__________

WORKOUT LOG

NAME:_________________________ GOALS:_________________________

EXERCISES	SETS	REPS	WT	REST	TIME	1 RM	NOTES

DATE:__________ WEIGHT:__________ SLEEP:__________ CALORIES:__________

EXERCISES	SETS	REPS	WT	REST	TIME	1 RM	NOTES

DATE:__________ WEIGHT:__________ SLEEP:__________ CALORIES:__________

EXERCISES	SETS	REPS	WT	REST	TIME	1 RM	NOTES

DATE:__________ WEIGHT:__________ SLEEP:__________ CALORIES:__________

EXERCISES	SETS	REPS	WT	REST	TIME	1 RM	NOTES

DATE:__________ WEIGHT:__________ SLEEP:__________ CALORIES:__________

EXERCISES	SETS	REPS	WT	REST	TIME	1 RM	NOTES

DATE:__________ WEIGHT:__________ SLEEP:__________ CALORIES:__________

WORKOUT LOG

NAME:_________________________   GOALS:_________________________

EXERCISES	SETS	REPS	WT	REST	TIME	1 RM	NOTES

DATE:_________   WEIGHT:_________   SLEEP:_________   CALORIES:_________

EXERCISES	SETS	REPS	WT	REST	TIME	1 RM	NOTES

DATE:_________   WEIGHT:_________   SLEEP:_________   CALORIES:_________

EXERCISES	SETS	REPS	WT	REST	TIME	1 RM	NOTES

DATE:_________   WEIGHT:_________   SLEEP:_________   CALORIES:_________

EXERCISES	SETS	REPS	WT	REST	TIME	1 RM	NOTES

DATE:_________   WEIGHT:_________   SLEEP:_________   CALORIES:_________

EXERCISES	SETS	REPS	WT	REST	TIME	1 RM	NOTES

DATE:_________   WEIGHT:_________   SLEEP:_________   CALORIES:_________

WORKOUT LOG

NAME:_________________________ GOALS:_________________________

EXERCISES	SETS	REPS	WT	REST	TIME	1 RM	NOTES

DATE:__________ WEIGHT:__________ SLEEP:__________ CALORIES:__________

EXERCISES	SETS	REPS	WT	REST	TIME	1 RM	NOTES

DATE:__________ WEIGHT:__________ SLEEP:__________ CALORIES:__________

EXERCISES	SETS	REPS	WT	REST	TIME	1 RM	NOTES

DATE:__________ WEIGHT:__________ SLEEP:__________ CALORIES:__________

EXERCISES	SETS	REPS	WT	REST	TIME	1 RM	NOTES

DATE:__________ WEIGHT:__________ SLEEP:__________ CALORIES:__________

EXERCISES	SETS	REPS	WT	REST	TIME	1 RM	NOTES

DATE:__________ WEIGHT:__________ SLEEP:__________ CALORIES:__________

WORKOUT LOG

NAME:_________________________   GOALS:_________________________

EXERCISES	SETS	REPS	WT	REST	TIME	1 RM	NOTES

DATE:__________   WEIGHT:__________   SLEEP:__________   CALORIES:__________

EXERCISES	SETS	REPS	WT	REST	TIME	1 RM	NOTES

DATE:__________   WEIGHT:__________   SLEEP:__________   CALORIES:__________

EXERCISES	SETS	REPS	WT	REST	TIME	1 RM	NOTES

DATE:__________   WEIGHT:__________   SLEEP:__________   CALORIES:__________

EXERCISES	SETS	REPS	WT	REST	TIME	1 RM	NOTES

DATE:__________   WEIGHT:__________   SLEEP:__________   CALORIES:__________

EXERCISES	SETS	REPS	WT	REST	TIME	1 RM	NOTES

DATE:__________   WEIGHT:__________   SLEEP:__________   CALORIES:__________

WORKOUT LOG

NAME:_________________________   GOALS:_________________________

EXERCISES	SETS	REPS	WT	REST	TIME	1 RM	NOTES

DATE:__________   WEIGHT:__________   SLEEP:__________   CALORIES:__________

EXERCISES	SETS	REPS	WT	REST	TIME	1 RM	NOTES

DATE:__________   WEIGHT:__________   SLEEP:__________   CALORIES:__________

EXERCISES	SETS	REPS	WT	REST	TIME	1 RM	NOTES

DATE:__________   WEIGHT:__________   SLEEP:__________   CALORIES:__________

EXERCISES	SETS	REPS	WT	REST	TIME	1 RM	NOTES

DATE:__________   WEIGHT:__________   SLEEP:__________   CALORIES:__________

EXERCISES	SETS	REPS	WT	REST	TIME	1 RM	NOTES

DATE:__________   WEIGHT:__________   SLEEP:__________   CALORIES:__________

WORKOUT LOG

NAME:________________________   GOALS:___________________

EXERCISES	SETS	REPS	WT	REST	TIME	1 RM	NOTES

DATE:__________   WEIGHT:__________   SLEEP:__________   CALORIES:__________

EXERCISES	SETS	REPS	WT	REST	TIME	1 RM	NOTES

DATE:__________   WEIGHT:__________   SLEEP:__________   CALORIES:__________

EXERCISES	SETS	REPS	WT	REST	TIME	1 RM	NOTES

DATE:__________   WEIGHT:__________   SLEEP:__________   CALORIES:__________

EXERCISES	SETS	REPS	WT	REST	TIME	1 RM	NOTES

DATE:__________   WEIGHT:__________   SLEEP:__________   CALORIES:__________

EXERCISES	SETS	REPS	WT	REST	TIME	1 RM	NOTES

DATE:__________   WEIGHT:__________   SLEEP:__________   CALORIES:__________

WORKOUT LOG

NAME:________________________ GOALS:________________________

EXERCISES	SETS	REPS	WT	REST	TIME	1 RM	NOTES

DATE:__________ WEIGHT:__________ SLEEP:__________ CALORIES:__________

EXERCISES	SETS	REPS	WT	REST	TIME	1 RM	NOTES

DATE:__________ WEIGHT:__________ SLEEP:__________ CALORIES:__________

EXERCISES	SETS	REPS	WT	REST	TIME	1 RM	NOTES

DATE:__________ WEIGHT:__________ SLEEP:__________ CALORIES:__________

EXERCISES	SETS	REPS	WT	REST	TIME	1 RM	NOTES

DATE:__________ WEIGHT:__________ SLEEP:__________ CALORIES:__________

EXERCISES	SETS	REPS	WT	REST	TIME	1 RM	NOTES

DATE:__________ WEIGHT:__________ SLEEP:__________ CALORIES:__________

WORKOUT LOG

NAME:________________________   GOALS:________________________

EXERCISES	SETS	REPS	WT	REST	TIME	1 RM	NOTES

DATE:__________   WEIGHT:__________   SLEEP:__________   CALORIES:__________

EXERCISES	SETS	REPS	WT	REST	TIME	1 RM	NOTES

DATE:__________   WEIGHT:__________   SLEEP:__________   CALORIES:__________

EXERCISES	SETS	REPS	WT	REST	TIME	1 RM	NOTES

DATE:__________   WEIGHT:__________   SLEEP:__________   CALORIES:__________

EXERCISES	SETS	REPS	WT	REST	TIME	1 RM	NOTES

DATE:__________   WEIGHT:__________   SLEEP:__________   CALORIES:__________

EXERCISES	SETS	REPS	WT	REST	TIME	1 RM	NOTES

DATE:__________   WEIGHT:__________   SLEEP:__________   CALORIES:__________

WORKOUT LOG

NAME:_____________________________ GOALS:_____________________________

EXERCISES	SETS	REPS	WT	REST	TIME	1 RM	NOTES

DATE:__________ WEIGHT:__________ SLEEP:__________ CALORIES:__________

EXERCISES	SETS	REPS	WT	REST	TIME	1 RM	NOTES

DATE:__________ WEIGHT:__________ SLEEP:__________ CALORIES:__________

EXERCISES	SETS	REPS	WT	REST	TIME	1 RM	NOTES

DATE:__________ WEIGHT:__________ SLEEP:__________ CALORIES:__________

EXERCISES	SETS	REPS	WT	REST	TIME	1 RM	NOTES

DATE:__________ WEIGHT:__________ SLEEP:__________ CALORIES:__________

EXERCISES	SETS	REPS	WT	REST	TIME	1 RM	NOTES

DATE:__________ WEIGHT:__________ SLEEP:__________ CALORIES:__________

WORKOUT LOG

NAME:________________________   GOALS:____________________

EXERCISES	SETS	REPS	WT	REST	TIME	1 RM	NOTES

DATE:__________   WEIGHT:__________   SLEEP:__________   CALORIES:__________

EXERCISES	SETS	REPS	WT	REST	TIME	1 RM	NOTES

DATE:__________   WEIGHT:__________   SLEEP:__________   CALORIES:__________

EXERCISES	SETS	REPS	WT	REST	TIME	1 RM	NOTES

DATE:__________   WEIGHT:__________   SLEEP:__________   CALORIES:__________

EXERCISES	SETS	REPS	WT	REST	TIME	1 RM	NOTES

DATE:__________   WEIGHT:__________   SLEEP:__________   CALORIES:__________

EXERCISES	SETS	REPS	WT	REST	TIME	1 RM	NOTES

DATE:__________   WEIGHT:__________   SLEEP:__________   CALORIES:__________

WORKOUT LOG

NAME:________________________   GOALS:________________________

EXERCISES	SETS	REPS	WT	REST	TIME	1 RM	NOTES

DATE:__________   WEIGHT:__________   SLEEP:__________   CALORIES:__________

EXERCISES	SETS	REPS	WT	REST	TIME	1 RM	NOTES

DATE:__________   WEIGHT:__________   SLEEP:__________   CALORIES:__________

EXERCISES	SETS	REPS	WT	REST	TIME	1 RM	NOTES

DATE:__________   WEIGHT:__________   SLEEP:__________   CALORIES:__________

EXERCISES	SETS	REPS	WT	REST	TIME	1 RM	NOTES

DATE:__________   WEIGHT:__________   SLEEP:__________   CALORIES:__________

EXERCISES	SETS	REPS	WT	REST	TIME	1 RM	NOTES

DATE:__________   WEIGHT:__________   SLEEP:__________   CALORIES:__________

WORKOUT LOG

NAME:________________________ GOALS:______________________

EXERCISES	SETS	REPS	WT	REST	TIME	1 RM	NOTES

DATE:__________ WEIGHT:__________ SLEEP:__________ CALORIES:__________

EXERCISES	SETS	REPS	WT	REST	TIME	1 RM	NOTES

DATE:__________ WEIGHT:__________ SLEEP:__________ CALORIES:__________

EXERCISES	SETS	REPS	WT	REST	TIME	1 RM	NOTES

DATE:__________ WEIGHT:__________ SLEEP:__________ CALORIES:__________

EXERCISES	SETS	REPS	WT	REST	TIME	1 RM	NOTES

DATE:__________ WEIGHT:__________ SLEEP:__________ CALORIES:__________

EXERCISES	SETS	REPS	WT	REST	TIME	1 RM	NOTES

DATE:__________ WEIGHT:__________ SLEEP:__________ CALORIES:__________

WORKOUT LOG

NAME:___________________________ GOALS:_______________________

EXERCISES	SETS	REPS	WT	REST	TIME	1 RM	NOTES

DATE:_________ WEIGHT:_________ SLEEP:_________ CALORIES:_________

EXERCISES	SETS	REPS	WT	REST	TIME	1 RM	NOTES

DATE:_________ WEIGHT:_________ SLEEP:_________ CALORIES:_________

EXERCISES	SETS	REPS	WT	REST	TIME	1 RM	NOTES

DATE:_________ WEIGHT:_________ SLEEP:_________ CALORIES:_________

EXERCISES	SETS	REPS	WT	REST	TIME	1 RM	NOTES

DATE:_________ WEIGHT:_________ SLEEP:_________ CALORIES:_________

EXERCISES	SETS	REPS	WT	REST	TIME	1 RM	NOTES

DATE:_________ WEIGHT:_________ SLEEP:_________ CALORIES:_________

WORKOUT LOG

NAME:_________________________ GOALS:_________________________

EXERCISES	SETS	REPS	WT	REST	TIME	1 RM	NOTES

DATE:__________ WEIGHT:__________ SLEEP:__________ CALORIES:__________

EXERCISES	SETS	REPS	WT	REST	TIME	1 RM	NOTES

DATE:__________ WEIGHT:__________ SLEEP:__________ CALORIES:__________

EXERCISES	SETS	REPS	WT	REST	TIME	1 RM	NOTES

DATE:__________ WEIGHT:__________ SLEEP:__________ CALORIES:__________

EXERCISES	SETS	REPS	WT	REST	TIME	1 RM	NOTES

DATE:__________ WEIGHT:__________ SLEEP:__________ CALORIES:__________

EXERCISES	SETS	REPS	WT	REST	TIME	1 RM	NOTES

DATE:__________ WEIGHT:__________ SLEEP:__________ CALORIES:__________

WORKOUT LOG

NAME:________________________ GOALS:________________________

EXERCISES	SETS	REPS	WT	REST	TIME	1 RM	NOTES

DATE:__________ WEIGHT:__________ SLEEP:__________ CALORIES:__________

EXERCISES	SETS	REPS	WT	REST	TIME	1 RM	NOTES

DATE:__________ WEIGHT:__________ SLEEP:__________ CALORIES:__________

EXERCISES	SETS	REPS	WT	REST	TIME	1 RM	NOTES

DATE:__________ WEIGHT:__________ SLEEP:__________ CALORIES:__________

EXERCISES	SETS	REPS	WT	REST	TIME	1 RM	NOTES

DATE:__________ WEIGHT:__________ SLEEP:__________ CALORIES:__________

EXERCISES	SETS	REPS	WT	REST	TIME	1 RM	NOTES

DATE:__________ WEIGHT:__________ SLEEP:__________ CALORIES:__________